The At-Home Guide to Safe Microneedling For Skin Rejuvenation

Karin Downes RE, CLT, FARM

Introduction

Discover the secrets to radiant and youthful skin with the at-home guide to safe microneedling for skin rejuvenation. This comprehensive book is your essential companion to mastering the art of microneedling in the comfort of your own home. Whether you're seeking to minimize fine Lines and wrinkles, fade acne scars, or improve overall texture, this guide provides you with the knowledge and techniques to achieve safe and effective microneedling results.

Inside this book, you will explore:

The science behind microneedling and how it rejuvenates the skin.

Choosing the right microneedling device and needle length for your specific skincare needs.

Step-by-step instructions on preparing your skin, performing microneedling, and post-treatment care.

Expert advice on optimizing results, managing potential risks, and achieving skin rejuvenation.

Disclaimer:

The information provided here is for educational purposes only and does not constitute legal or medical advice. before engaging in at-home microneedling, it is essential to consult with a qualified healthcare professional or dermatologist to assess the suitability of the procedure for your skin type and condition. By choosing to perform at-home microneedling, you accept all Associated risks and liabilities. this disclaimer absolves any parties involved in providing this information from any legal responsibility for any adverse effects or Consequences resulting from the at home micro-needling procedure. additionally, it is recommended to carefully read and adhere to all safety instructions provided by the microneedling device manufacturer

Table of Contents

Chapter 1. What happens when you microneedle

Chapter 2. Benefits of microneedling as a Skin Care Treatment

Chapter 3. Choosing the right device

Chapter 4. Preparing for at home micronneedling

Chapter 5. Performing at home microneedling

Chapter 6. Results and follow-up treatments

CHAPTER 1

What happens when you microneedle?

When microneedling is performed, the micro-injuries created in the skin trigger a cascade of cellular responses. The initial injury causes the release of growth factors and cytokines, which attract immune cells to the site of injury. These immune cells help remove damaged tissue and stimulate collagen and elastin production. Collagen is a protein essential for skin strength and elasticity, while elastin provides skin with its ability to stretch and bounce back. The production of these proteins helps to repair and rejuvenate the skin, reducing the appearance of fine lines, wrinkles, and scars. Additionally, the microneedling process increases blood flow to the treated area, delivering oxygen and nutrients to support skin regeneration. Overall, the scientific reaction in the skin when microneedling includes increased collagen and elastin production, improved skin texture and firmness, enhanced skin healing, and a rejuvenated appearance.

What areas can be treated with microneedling?

Microneedling can be used to treat a variety of skin concerns on different areas of the body. Some common areas that can be treated with microneedling include:

Face: Microneedling is commonly used on the face to improve skin texture, reduce wrinkles and fine lines, minimize pores, and improve overall skin tone and firmness.

Neck: Microneedling can help to tighten and rejuvenate the skin on the neck, reducing the appearance of sagging skin and fine lines.

Decolletage: Microneedling can be used to treat the chest area, known as decolletage, to improve skin texture, reduce sun damage, and address wrinkles and fine lines.

Hands: Microneedling can also be used on the hands to improve skin texture, reduce age spots, and rejuvenate the appearance of the skin.

Scars: Microneedling can help to improve the appearance of acne scars, surgical scars, and other types of scars by promoting collagen production and skin regeneration.

Stretch marks: Microneedling can also reduce the appearance of stretch marks by stimulating collagen production and improving skin texture.

The face is typically divided into three main regions: the forehead, the midface (which includes the eyes, nose, and cheeks), and the lower face (which includes the mouth, chin, jawline, and the upper portion of the face, including the hairline and the area above the eyebrows).

The midface contains the eyes, which are positioned in the center of the face, with the nose below and the cheeks on either side.

The lower face includes the mouth, which is located below the nose, the chin at the bottom of the face, and the jawline which extends from the chin to the ears on either side.

It's important to consult with a trained and experienced skincare professional to determine the most appropriate treatment plan for your specific skin concerns and desired outcome

CHAPTER 2

Benefits of Micro-Needling as a skin care treatment include:

Collagen production: The micro-injuries caused by microneedling stimulate the skin to produce new collagen, which helps to improve skin texture, reduce the appearance of fine lines and wrinkles, and enhance skin firmness.

Skin rejuvenation: Microneedling promotes skin cell regeneration and turnover, leading to a refreshed and rejuvenated complexion.

Improved skincare product absorption: The micro-channels created by micro-needling allow for better penetration of skincare products, increasing their effectiveness in delivering beneficial ingredients to the skin.

Reduction of scars and hyperpigmentation: Microneedling can help minimize the appearance of acne scars, surgical scars, and hyperpigmentation by promoting collagen production and skin regeneration.

Treatment of skin conditions: Microneedling is used to address various skin concerns such as acne, enlarged pores, and uneven skin tone.

Cost-Effective Option: At home, microneedling.Can be a more affordable alternative to professional treatments, offering convenience and flexibility for regular use.

When beginning your at-home microneedling treatment, it is essential to have realistic expectations regarding the results you can achieve. Here are some factors to consider when setting expectations for at-home microneedling results:

Gradual Improvement: Microneedling is a gradual process that stimulates collagen production and skin regeneration over time. Results may not be immediately noticeable, and multiple treatment sessions are usually required to achieve significant improvements in skin texture, tone, and appearance.

Skin Concerns: The extent of improvement in various skin concerns, such as wrinkles, acne scars, hyperpigmentation, and fine lines, will vary based on your skin type, the depth of the treatment, and the consistency of the microneedling regimen. Some concerns may show more visible improvement than others.

Skin Type and Condition: Individuals with different skin types and conditions may respond differently to microneedling treatment. Factors such as skin elasticity, sun damage, and underlying skin conditions can influence the effectiveness of microneedling and the visible results achieved.

Consistency and Maintenance: As recommended by skin care professionals, consistent and regular microneedling sessions are crucial for achieving optimal results. Additionally, following a proper skincare routine, protecting the skin from sun exposure, and avoiding harsh products post-treatment can help maintain and enhance the results of microneedling.

Professional Guidance: While at-home microneedling can be effective, consulting with a skincare professional or dermatologist can provide personalized recommendations, guidance, and insights on how to maximize the benefits of microneedling based on your skin concerns and goals.

Realistic Expectations: It is important to have realistic expectations about the results of at-home microneedling. While microneedling can improve skin texture, firmness, and overall appearance, it may not completely eliminate deep wrinkles, severe scars, or advanced signs of aging. Setting realistic goals ensures satisfaction with the results achieved through microneedling treatment.

By understanding these factors and setting realistic expectations for at-home microneedling results, you can have a clear understanding of the potential benefits and outcomes of the treatment, allowing you to track progress, make informed decisions, and enjoy the improvements to your skin over time.

At-home microneedling can offer several benefits for skin rejuvenation and improvement, but it also comes with certain risks that need to be considered. Below is a discussion of the benefits and risks of at-home microneedling.

Benefits of At-Home Microneedling:

Skin Rejuvenation: At-home microneedling can stimulate collagen production, improving skin texture, firmness, and elasticity.

Reduction of Fine Lines and Wrinkles: Microneedling can help reduce the appearance of fine lines and wrinkles by promoting skin regeneration.

Improved Absorption of Skincare Products: The microchannels created by microneedling can enhance the penetration and effectiveness of skincare products, maximizing their benefits.

Treatment of Scars and Hyperpigmentation: At-home microneedling can reduce the appearance of acne scars, hyperpigmentation, and other skin discolorations.

Cost-Effective Option: At-home microneedling can be a more affordable alternative to professional treatments, offering convenience and flexibility for regular use.

Risks of At-Home Microneedling:

Skin Irritation and Sensitivity: Improper technique or using a device with needles that are too long can cause skin irritation, redness, and sensitivity.

Infection: Using nonsterile or low-quality microneedling devices can increase the risk of infection and skin damage.

Increased Sensitivity to Sun: Microneedling can temporarily increase skin sensitivity to sunlight, making it crucial to use adequate sun protection.

Exacerbation of Skin Conditions: At-home microneedling may worsen certain skin conditions, such as eczema, psoriasis, or active acne.

Risk of Bruising or Bleeding: Using excessive pressure or incorrect needle lengths can result in bruising or minor bleeding during microneedling.

Following proper guidelines, hygiene practices, and safety precautions is important when performing at-home microneedling to minimize the risks and maximize the benefits. Consulting with a skincare professional before starting at-home microneedling can provide tailored advice, ensure safe use of the equipment being used, and help address any concerns or skin conditions that may affect the treatment outcomes. By understanding both the benefits and risks of at-home microneedling individuals can make informed decisions and achieve positive results in their skin care routine.

Differences between professional microneedling and at-home microneedling

Professional microneedling and at-home microneedling are two methods of skin treatment that involve the use of microneedling devices to create controlled micro-injuries in the skin. While they both aim to stimulate collagen production. While at-home devices come with instructions, the user may not properly microneedle correctly to improve skin texture, There are significant differences between the two approaches. Here are some key distinctions:

Skill and Expertise:

Professional Microneedling: Professional microneedling is typically performed by trained skincare professionals, such as dermatologists or estheticians, who have the knowledge and experience to customize the treatment based on individual skin concerns and conditions.

At-Home Microneedling: At-home microneedling is self-administered by individuals without professional supervision, and it does not require the same level of expertise or understanding of proper technique as a trained professional.

2. **Device and Needle Quality:**

Professional Microneedling: Professional clinics use medical-grade microneedling devices with high-quality needles that are sterile and carefully maintained to ensure safety and effectiveness.

At-Home Microneedling: At-home microneedling devices vary in quality, and if not used correctly, lower-quality or unsterile devices may lead to skin irritation, infection, or other complications.

3. **Treatment Depth and Intensity: Professional Microneedling:** Professional microneedling uses longer needles to reach deeper layers of the skin, allowing for more intensive treatments that target specific skin concerns.

At-Home Microneedling: At-home microneedling devices typically have shorter needles and may not penetrate the skin as deeply as professional treatments. This difference in treatment depth may affect the level of results achieved.

Results and Safety:

Professional microneedling: Treatments are often more effective and provide consistent, controlled results under the supervision of a trained professional. The risk of complications is minimized in a clinical setting.

At-Home Microneedling: While at-home microneedling can offer convenience and flexibility for regular treatments, it can also increase the risk of user error, skin damage, or adverse reactions if proper hygiene practices and techniques are not followed

Overall Experience:

Professional Microneedling: Professional microneedling treatments offer a spa-like experience, focusing on comfort, safety, and customized care tailored to individual needs

At-home microneedling: can be positive and rewarding for those who prioritize safety, adhere to proper techniques, and manage expectations regarding results and potential discomfort. By staying informed, following guidelines, and seeking professional guidance when needed, individuals can enjoy the benefits of microneedling while minimizing risks and promoting healthy, radiant skin.

CHAPTER 3

Choosing the right microneedling device

When choosing a microneedling device for at-home use, there are several factors to consider to ensure safety, efficacy, and optimal results. Here are some key points to keep in mind when selecting the right microneedling device:

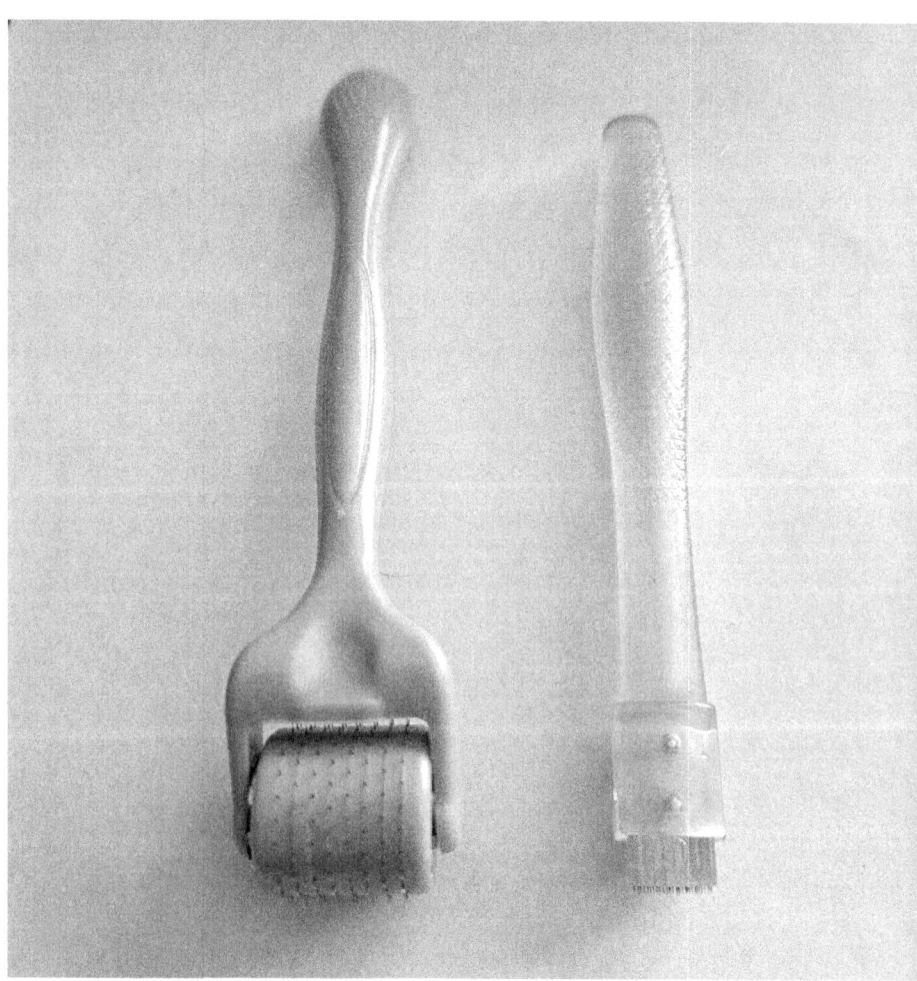

Needle Length: Choose a microneedling device with an appropriate needle length based on your skin concerns and treatment goals. Shorter needles (.02mm to .05mm) are typically recommended for at-home use to minimize the risk of injury and ensure safe treatment.

Needle Quality: Opt for a microneedling device with high-quality, medical-grade stainless steel needles that are sharp, durable, and sterile. Poor-quality needles can cause skin irritation, uneven results, or breakage during treatment.

Needle Type: Consider the type of microneedling device that best suits your needs. Dermarollers feature a roller with needles attached to a wheel while microneedling pens have a motorized pen-like design with disposable needle cartridges. The author does not recommend motorized devices for at-home use. Choose a device type that you feel comfortable using, and that fits your treatment preferences.

Brand Reputation: Research reputable brands known for producing high-quality microneedling devices that are safe and efficacious. Reading customer reviews and seeking recommendations from skincare professionals can help you make an informed decision.

Safety Features: Look for microneedling devices with safety features, such as quality stainless needles of the appropriate length. These features contribute to a safer and more effective microneedling experience.

Budget: Consider your budget when choosing a microneedling device. While quality devices may come at a higher price point, investing in a reliable and safe device can ensure better results and reduce the risk of complications.

Consultation: If you are uncertain about which microneedling device to choose, consider consulting with a skincare professional or dermatologist for recommendations based on your skin type, concerns, and treatment goals. By considering these factors and conducting thorough research, you can select the right microneedling device for at-home skin care treatment, ensuring safety, efficacy, and optimal results. It is important to follow the manufacturer's instructions and guidelines for proper use and maintenance of the microneedling device to achieve the desired skin improvements.

CHAPTER 4

Preparing for at home Microneedling

Preparing for at-home microneedling is essential to ensure a safe and effective treatment. Here are some important steps to consider when getting ready for microneedling at home:

Research and Education:

Familiarize yourself with the microneedling process, benefits, and potential risks.

Read the manufacturer's instructions for the micro needling device you will be using. For additional guidance, watch instructional videos or seek advice from skincare professionals.

2, Skin Assessment: Evaluate your skin type, concerns, and areas you wish to target with micro needling. Note any existing skin conditions, scars, or sensitivities that may affect the treatment.

Choose the right microneedling device: Select a high-quality microneedling device with an appropriate needle length for at-home use. Ensure the device is clean, sterilized, and in good working condition before each treatment. If you accidentally drop it or bump in on anything, do not use it as the needles can barb.

Prepare Your Skin: Cleanse your skin thoroughly to remove makeup, dirt, and debris. To reduce the risk of infection, disinfect the treatment area with an alcohol swab.

Numbing Cream (optional) If using, use only a 5% lidocaine cream. You would only need it at .05 depth. You would apply it generously and leave it on for 20 minutes. You don't need topical for .02 mm to .03mm

I recommend don't use longer than 0.5 mm. Start with a .02 mm or 0.25mm.

7. Set Up Your Treatment Space. Choose a clean and well-lit area with a flat surface to perform the microneedling treatment. Have all necessary supplies, including the microneedling device, skincare products, and clean towels, within reach.

8. Follow a Post-Treatment Plan:

Plan your post-treatment skincare routine, including gentle cleansers, hydrating serums, and moisturizers to soothe and protect the skin after microneedling.

Avoid harsh skincare products, direct sun exposure, and intense physical activities immediately following the treatment. Should you have any concerns or questions about at-home microneedling, consider consulting with a skincare professional or dermatologist for personalized advice and recommendations.

By taking these steps to prepare for at-home microneedling, you can ensure a safe and successful treatment experience. Following proper pretreatment guidelines and maintaining good skincare practices will help optimize the results of microneedling and promote skin health and rejuvenatioChapter 5

Chapter 5

Performing Microneedling at home

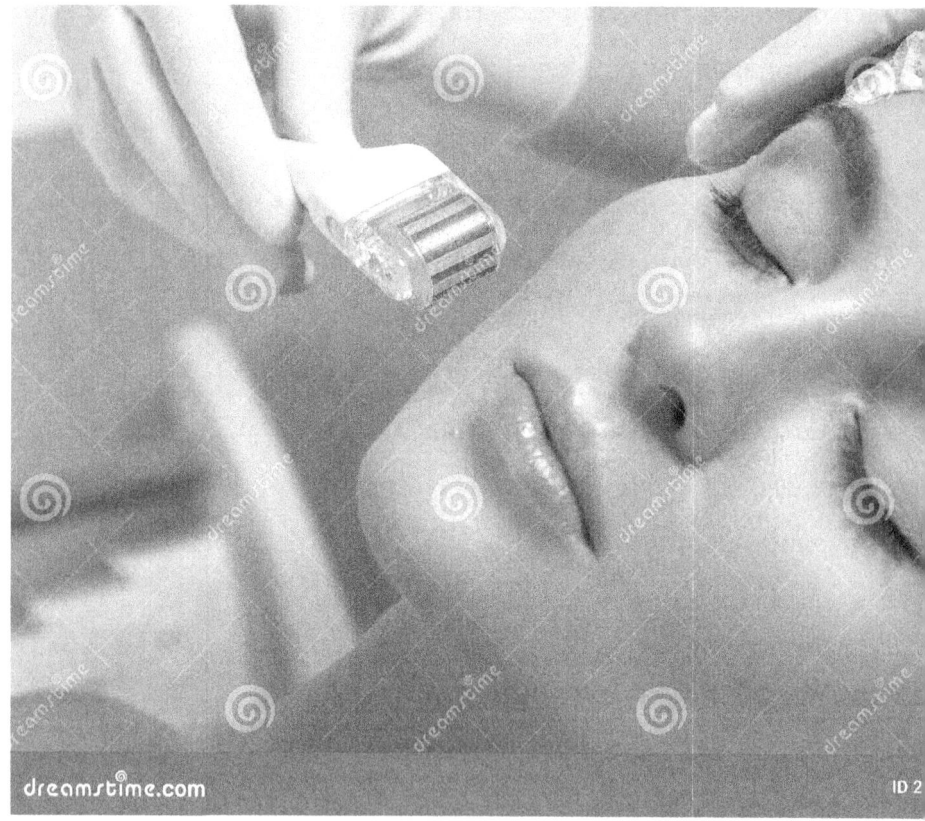

Performing microneedling at home requires careful preparation, proper technique, and post-treatment care to ensure safe and effective results. Here is a step-by-step guide on how to perform microneedling at home:

Cleanse Your Skin: Start by washing your face with a gentle cleanser to remove any makeup, dirt, and bacteria. Pat your skin dry with a clean towel to ensure it is completely clean before microneedling.

Disinfect Your Microneedling Device: Disinfect the microneedling device by soaking it in rubbing alcohol for at least 10 minutes. Rinse the device with warm water and let it air dry before use to ensure it is clean and sterile.

Prepare the Treatment Area: Choose the area on your skin that you wish to treat with micro needling. Section off smaller parts of the treatment area to ensure thorough coverage and consistent results. Use only sterile saline or high-molecular-weight Hyaluronic acid on the skin.

Perform Microneedling: Hold the microneedling device at a 90-degree angle to your skin and gently roll or stamp it over the treatment area in vertical, horizontal, and diagonal directions. Apply light to moderate pressure but avoid pressing too hard on the skin to prevent discomfort or injury. Never roll back and forth in the same roll. Upwards sideways, diagonal, and diagonal. Continue microneedling in the desired areas, ensuring even coverage and avoiding sensitive areas like the eyes and lips.

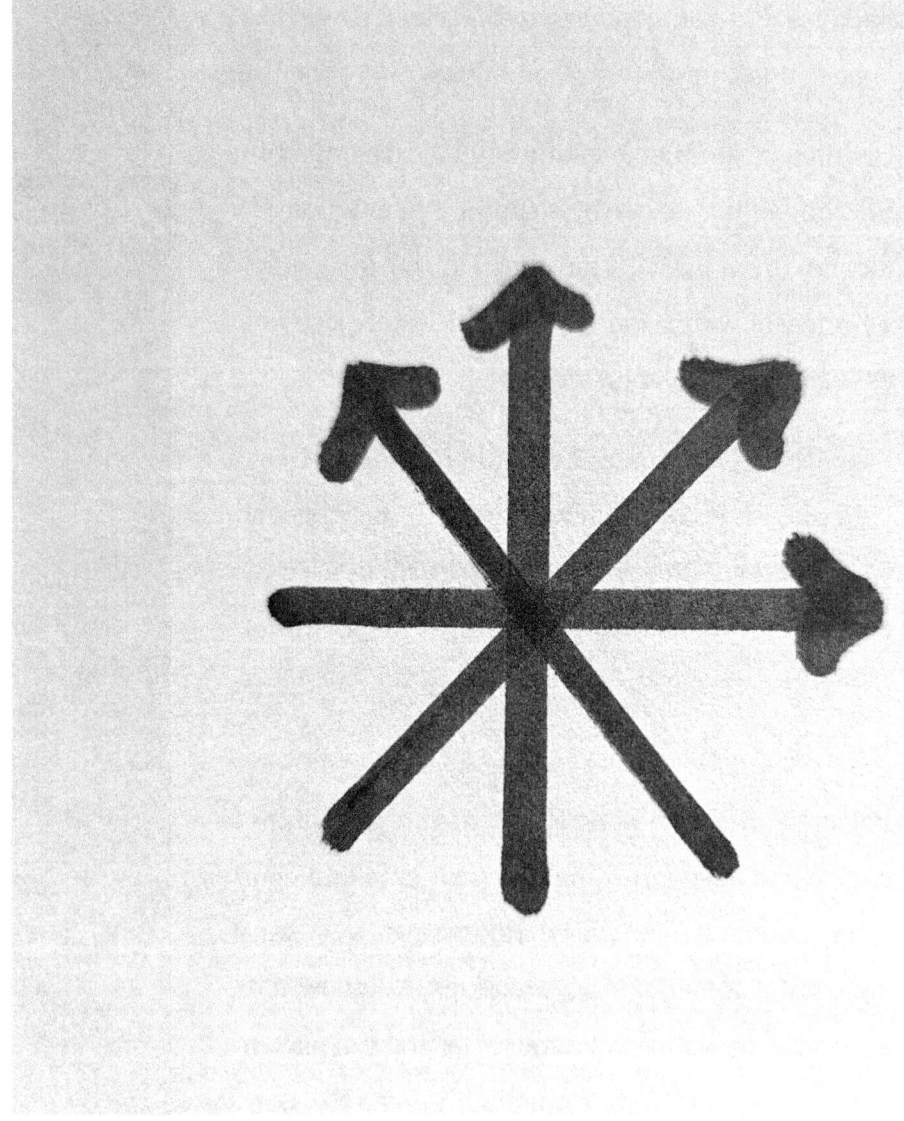

Do a small section at a time Connect each section.

5. Apply Hyaluronic Acid or a hydrating moisturizer to the treated skin to promote healing and nourishment. If you don't have access to a professional skincare line, I recommend either

organic grape seed oil, organic coconut oil, or organic linseed oil afterward.

To prevent irritation, avoid using harsh skincare products, exfoliants, or makeup immediately after microneedling. Protect your skin from direct sunlight and wear sunscreen with SPF to prevent UV damage. I recommend going to the baby department and getting a high-SPF baby sunscreen with no chemicals. Do not apply it on the day of needling; wait until the following day.

Clean and Store Your Microneedling Device:

After use, rinse the microneedling device with warm water and mild soap to remove any residue. Disinfect the device again by soaking it in rubbing alcohol before storing it in a clean, dry place. The device may also be sanitized by taking a denture tablet, placing it in a glass of water with a cotton round at the bottom to protect it, filling it with water, and leaving it in there until the water goes clear. then you can put it back in your case and store it till the next treatment.

The Follow-Up and Maintenance:

Wait for a few weeks between microneedling sessions to allow your skin to heal and regenerate.

Monitor your skin for any redness, irritation, or adverse reactions and adjust your microneedling routine as needed.

It is essential to follow these steps carefully, adhere to proper hygiene practices, and consult with a skincare professional if you have any concerns or questions about performing microneedling at home. By following these guidelines, you can achieve safe and effective results in

Post-treatment care is crucial after performing microneedling at home to ensure proper healing, minimize the risk of complications, and optimize the results of the treatment. Here are some essential post-treatment care tips for at-home microneedling:

Avoid Sun Exposure: After microneedling, protect your skin from direct sunlight by wearing a broad-spectrum sunscreen with at least SPF 30. Sun exposure can increase the risk of skin damage and hinder the healing process.

Hydrate Your Skin: Use a gentle, hydrating serum or moisturizer to keep your skin moisturized and prevent dryness. Look for products with soothing ingredients like aloe vera, hyaluronic acid, or vitamin E to nourish the skin post-treatment. Stay away from parabens and harsh chemicals in your skincare line.

Avoid Harsh Skincare Products: Avoid using harsh or chemical-laden skincare products immediately after micro needling. Stick to gentle, non-irritating products to avoid further sensitizing the skin.

Keep Your Skin Clean: Maintain good hygiene by cleansing your skin with a gentle cleanser to remove bacteria, dirt, and debris. Avoid harsh scrubbing or exfoliation for a few days following the treatment.

After microneedling, monitor your skin for any signs of redness, irritation, swelling, or infection. Contact a healthcare professional if you experience persistent or severe symptoms. Stay Hydrated: Drink plenty of water to keep your skin hydrated from the inside out. Proper hydration is essential for skin healing and regeneration after microneedling.

Avoid Makeup and Sweat: Refrain from applying makeup or engaging in activities that cause excessive sweating for the first 24-48 hours post-treatment. Give your skin time to recover without clogging pores or aggravating sensitive

Monitor Your Skin:

Follow a Gentle Skincare Routine: Stick to a simple and gentle skincare routine in the days following microneedling. Opt for products that are fragrance-free, hypoallergenic, and suited for sensitive skin to avoid further irritation.

Be Patient: Allow your skin time to heal and regenerate after microneedling. Results may take several weeks to become noticeable, so be patient and consistent with your post-treatment care routine.

By following these post-treatment care tips, you can promote healing, reduce the risk of complications, and enhance the effects of at-home microneedling. If you have any concerns or experience unusual reactions, seek guidance from a skincare professional or dermatologist.

Risks and considerations

At-home microneedling can be an effective skin treatment, but it also carries certain risks and considerations that should be taken into account before proceeding with the procedure. Here are some common risks and considerations for at-home microneedling:

Infection: Using unsterile microneedling devices or improperly sanitizing the skin before treatment can increase the risk of infection. It is essential to disinfect the device and thoroughly cleanse the skin to minimize the likelihood of bacterial contamination.

Skin Irritation: Microneedling can cause redness, swelling, and skin irritation, especially if the treatment is too aggressive or if the skin is not properly prepared. To prevent skin irritation, following proper techniques and avoiding excessive pressure is crucial.

3. Hyperpigmentation: Individuals with darker skin tones are at a higher risk of developing post-inflammatory hyperpigmentation after microneedling. It is important to consult with a skincare professional to determine the appropriate needle length and treatment intensity for your skin type.

4. Scarring: Improper micro needling technique, using a device with overly long needles, or treating active acne or open wounds can result in scarring. To minimize the risk of scarring, careful consideration should be given to the depth and frequency of the treatment.

5. Allergic Reactions: Some individuals may be allergic to certain skincare products or ingredients used before or after microneedling. Perform a patch test with products to check for sensitivity and consult with a dermatologist if you have any concerns.

6. Exacerbation of Skin Conditions: Microneedling may worsen certain skin conditions, such as eczema, psoriasis, rosacea, or active acne. Individuals with underlying skin conditions should consult with a healthcare professional before attempting microneedling at home. I Recommend not ever needle over any active irritated skin conditions, such as psoriasis, eczema, raised moles, or anything you're not sure what it is. If in doubt, don't treat it!

7. Needle Misuse: Using an inappropriate needle length or applying excessive pressure during microneedling can lead to skin damage, pain, or uneven results. Proper knowledge of the device and technique is crucial to minimize the risk of needle misuse.

8. Prolonged Healing Time: Microneedling may result in redness, swelling, and slight discomfort post-treatment, requiring a few days for the skin to fully recover. Allow for adequate healing time and

follow post-treatment care instructions to support the skin's recovery process.

9. If you've ever had a cold sore outbreak it would be advised to take a prophylactic antiviral before needling. Nerve-ending aggravations around the mouth can result in the break out of a cold sore if you have the virus in your system.

Before attempting microneedling at home, it is advisable to consult with a skincare professional or dermatologist to assess your skin's suitability for the Results and follow-up.

Aer performing at-home microneedling, it is important to understand the expected results, follow-up care, and potential outcomes to ensure optimal skincare benefits. Here is a guide to the results, follow-up, and ongoing care after at-home microneedling:

Expected Results:

Improved Skin Texture: Microneedling stimulates collagen production, leading to smoother and firmer skin texture over time.

Reduction of Fine Lines and Wrinkles: The treatment can help minimize the appearance of fine lines and wrinkles, resulting in a more youthful complexion.

4. Scar Reduction: Microneedling may improve the appearance of acne scars, surgery scars, and other types of skin blemishes.

6. Hyperpigmentation Improvement: The procedure can help lighten dark spots and hyperpigmentation for a more even skin tone.

Enhanced Product Absorption: Microneedling creates microchannels in the skin, allowing skincare products to penetrate more effectively for enhanced benefits.

Follow-Up Care:

Moisturize and Hydrate: Apply a hydrating serum or moisturizer to keep the skin well-hydrated and promote healing.

Sun Protection: Use a broad-spectrum sunscreen daily to protect the skin fax rom UV damage and prevent post-inflammatory hyperpigmentation.

Gentle Skincare: For a few days after treatment, stick to a gentle skincare routine and avoid harsh exfoliants or active ingredients.

Monitor Skin Reactions: Check your skin for redness, irritation, or adverse reactions, and contact a professional if necessary.

Follow Post-Treatment Instructions: For optimal results, adhere to the recommended post-treatment instructions provided by the manufacturer or skincare professional.

Expected Side Effects:

Redness and Swelling: Mild redness and swelling are common post-microneedling and usually subside within a few days.

Sensitivity: The treated skin may be more sensitive after the procedure, so be gentle with your skincare routine.

Dryness: Some dryness may occur due to the skin's healing process; make sure to keep the skin well moisturized.

CHAPTER 6

Results and Follow-Up Treatments:

The frequency of at-home microneedling treatments can vary depending on your skin concerns and goals.

Allow sufficient time between treatments. If you use a .02 mm to a .03 you could needle daily. If you are using a .05 mm (generally 4-6 weeks) to allow your skin to fully recover and see the effects of the previous session.

Consistency is key to achieving and maintaining results with microneedling, so regular follow-up treatments may be recommended for continued improvement.

Professional Consultation:

Consider seeking a professional consultation with a skincare expert or dermatologist to assess your skin condition, address any concerns, and receive personalized recommendations for at-home microneedling.

Professionals can provide guidance on the appropriate needle length, treatment intensity, and skincare products to maximize the benefits of microneedling.

By following these guidelines for post-treatment care, expectations, and follow-up, you can enhance the results of at-home microneedling and maintain healthy, rejuvenated skin over time. It is essential to be patient, consistent, and attentive to your skin's needs to achieve the desired outcomes and enjoy the long-term benefits of microneedling. If you have any questions or experience persistent skin reactions, consult a skin care professional or dermatologist for further guidance and support.

In conclusion, microneedling at home can be a beneficial skin treatment when done safely and effectively. To ensure optimal results and minimize risks, here is a summary of key points for performing microneedling at home:

Choose the Right Microneedling Device:

Select a high-quality microneedling device with an appropriate needle length for at-home use.

Ensure the device is clean, sterile, and in good working condition before each treatment.

Skin Preparation:

Cleanse your skin thoroughly to remove dirt, makeup, and bacteria.

Disinfect the treatment area with an alcohol swab to minimize the risk of infection

Performing Microneedling

Hold the device at a 90-degree angle and apply gentle pressure while rolling or stamping over the skin.

Avoid excessive pressure or aggressive treatment to prevent skin irritation or damage.

Post-Treatment Care:

Avoid sun exposure and wear sunscreen to protect your skin.

Use soothing serums or moisturizers to hydrate and nourish the skin.

Follow a gentle skincare routine and avoid harsh products post-treatment.

Expected Results:

Microneedling is expected to improve skin texture, reduce fine lines and wrinkles, reduce scars, and improve hyperpigmentation.

Conclusion

By following these key points for safety and effective microneedling at home, you can achieve optimal results, promote skin health, and minimize the risks associated with the treatment. Prioritize proper preparation, skin care, and post-treatment care to ensure a successful at-home microneedling experience. Remember, consistency, patience, and attention to your skin's needs are essential for long-term skin rejuvenation and maintenance through microneedling. If you have any concerns or questions, seek professional guidance to support your skincare journey.

If any of the information in this book was beneficial to you, please go to Amazon and leave me a favorable review.

Resources

The Concise Guide to Dermal Needling by

Dr. Lance Setterfield

www.https://Dreamtime.com

About the Author

Karin Downes started in the beauty field in 1981 performing electrolysis treatments. She worked for doctors from 1981 to 1983 who invented laser hair removal, established protocols, and performed laser treatments. Karin went on to become a licensed nail technician. She then branched out to perform permanent cosmetics. She is a Board-certified, Certified Master and Certified Trainer in Howell Michigan. In 1999 she heard about a new treatment called Multitrepanic Collagen Actuation. She traveled to California to train under Dr Kristanne Matzek. Karin learned how to revise scars, wrinkles, acne scars, and burn scars. when Karin started to perform these procedures, there were less than five people in the whole country doing this. " We were having a hard time getting it into the medical community's hands because they wanted someone to agree to do a punch biopsy in the areas that we were revising to prove that it really worked." Nobody wanted to have a scar created from a punch biopsy when they were trying to get rid of scars. Once Dr. Des Fernandes spoke about it at a plastic surgery conference then it became documented as his Medical research and the treatment started gaining in popularity. Upon speaking to Dr Des Fernandes, he gave Karin his permission to utilize his research so she could speak about it at a conference in Las Vegas for the Society of Permanent Cosmetic Professionals in 2005. Upon speaking about it, and showing the research as to why it worked, it began to gain popularity across the country. When Dr. Lance Setterfield, the author of the book "The Concise Guide to Dermal Needling," had his first training in the United States for Dermal Needling, Karin trained with him to learn every aspect she could about it. Karin has treated clients all around the world for wrinkle reduction, acne scar revision, and simple scar revision.

Karin went on to become a New World Practitioner and a Whole Life Coach, training under Dr Darryl Wolfe, who is known as the Doc of Detox performing treatments for the reduction of scar tissue, calcification, and crystallization in the body. She then went on to become a Certified Lumia Science Technique Specialist, performing light therapy for healing tissue.

Karin presently owns the American Institute of Permanent Beauty and Rejuvenation where she performs and teaches permanent cosmetics and skin rejuvenation.

She can be reached for professional advice at Karin@aipbr.com.

Printed in Dunstable, United Kingdom

75305406R00030